BLOOD PRESSURE UNDER CONTROL

Monitor Vital Numbers, Spot Trends, and Make Smart Choices for a Healthier Life

DigiMedical

This publication is intended for personal use and general information purposes only. It does not constitute medical advice, diagnosis, or treatment. Always consult a licensed healthcare provider for medical concerns. The publisher and author disclaim any liability for actions taken based on the contents of this book.

PUBLISHED BY: ADALYNN JAMES PUBLISHING
Blue Ash, OH 45242
www.adalynnjames.com

ADALYNN JAMES

Understanding Your Blood Pressure: What the Numbers Mean

Blood pressure is one of the most important indicators of your heart health. This page will help you understand what your readings mean and why tracking them daily can save your life.

What is Blood Pressure?

Blood pressure is the force of blood pushing against the walls of your arteries. It's recorded as two numbers:

- Systolic Pressure: The top number. It measures the pressure when your heart beats and pumps blood.
- Diastolic Pressure: The bottom number. It measures the pressure when your heart is at rest between beats.

Both numbers are important. One or both being too high can put you at risk of heart disease, stroke, kidney damage, and more.

How Do You Know If You Have High Blood Pressure?

You may not feel any symptoms—that's why it's often called the "silent killer." The only way to know is to check it regularly.

Common risk factors include:

- Family history
- Poor diet (especially salty foods)
- Lack of exercise
- Smoking
- Stress
- Certain health conditions

What is a Healthy Blood Pressure?

According to the American Heart Association (AHA), here are the current guidelines:

Blood Pressure Category	Systolic Top Number	Diastolic Bottom Number
Normal	Less than 120	Less than 80
Elevated	120 - 129	Less than 80
High Blood Pressure (Stage 1)	130 - 139	80-89
High Blood Pressure (Stage 2)	140 or higher	90 or higher
Hypertensive Crisis (Seek Emergency Care)	Higher than 180	Higher than 120

A hypertensive crisis requires immediate medical attention.

What About Low Blood Pressure?

Low blood pressure (hypotension) is usually defined as a reading below 90/60. While it may not always be dangerous, symptoms can signal an underlying issue.

Signs of Low Blood Pressure:

- Dizziness or lightheadedness
- Fainting
- Blurred vision
- Cold, clammy, or pale skin
- Fatigue
- Nausea

When to Seek Emergency Help

Seek immediate medical attention if your low blood pressure is accompanied by:

- Fainting or loss of consciousness
- Chest pain or difficulty breathing
- A weak, rapid pulse
- Confusion or trouble speaking
- Severe dizziness or inability to stand

These may signal shock, heart issues, or serious blood loss.

Important:

- If something feels wrong, don't wait. It's better to be safe and get help. Call 911 or go to the ER.

Why This Logbook Matters:

Tracking your blood pressure at home helps:

- Identify patterns and triggers (like stress or salty meals)
- Share accurate information with your doctor
- Make better choices about food, exercise, and medication

Write your results daily. Bring this log to your appointments. You're taking control—and that's a powerful step toward better health.

Keep Going—You've Got This!

- This logbook is for YOU. Use it to stay on track and take charge of your health.
- Focus on progress, not perfection. Small daily efforts add up.
- Be proud of yourself. You're doing something important for your body and your future.

"Small steps lead to big results. Keep moving forward."

— DigiMedical, by Adalynn James Publishing

Blood Pressure Log

Month __________ **Year** __________ **Weight** __________

Date	Time	Blood Pressure		Pulse Heart Rate	Medication
		Systolic Top Number	Diastolic Bottom Number		
		/			
		/			
		/			
		/			
		/			
		/			
		/			
		/			
		/			
		/			
		/			

Notes

Blood Pressure Log

Month ____________ Year __________ Weight _________

Date	Time	Blood Pressure		Pulse	Medication
		Systolic Top Number	**Diastolic** Bottom Number	**Pulse** Heart Rate	
		/			
		/			
		/			
		/			
		/			
		/			
		/			
		/			

Blood Pressure Category	Systolic Top Number	Diastolic Bottom Number
Normal	Less than 120	Less than 80
Elevated	120 - 129	Less than 80
High Blood Pressure (Stage 1)	130 - 139	80-89
High Blood Pressure (Stage 2)	140 or higher	90 or higher
Hypertensive Crisis (Seek Emergency Care)	Higher than 180	Higher than 120

Blood Pressure Log

Month ____________ **Year** __________ **Weight** _________

Date	Time	Blood Pressure: Systolic Top Number	Blood Pressure: Diastolic Bottom Number	Pulse Heart Rate	Medication
		/			
		/			
		/			
		/			
		/			
		/			
		/			
		/			
		/			
		/			
		/			

Notes

Blood Pressure Log

Month ____________ Year __________ Weight _________

Date	Time	Blood Pressure: Systolic Top Number	Blood Pressure: Diastolic Bottom Number	Pulse Heart Rate	Medication
		/			
		/			
		/			
		/			
		/			
		/			
		/			
		/			

Blood Pressure Category	Systolic Top Number	Diastolic Bottom Number
Normal	Less than 120	Less than 80
Elevated	120 - 129	Less than 80
High Blood Pressure (Stage 1)	130 - 139	80-89
High Blood Pressure (Stage 2)	140 or higher	90 or higher
Hypertensive Crisis (Seek Emergency Care)	Higher than 180	Higher than 120

Blood Pressure Log

Month ____________ **Year** __________ **Weight** ________

Date	Time	Blood Pressure: Systolic Top Number	Blood Pressure: Diastolic Bottom Number	Pulse Heart Rate	Medication
		/			
		/			
		/			
		/			
		/			
		/			
		/			
		/			
		/			
		/			
		/			

Notes

Blood Pressure Log

Month ____________ Year __________ Weight _________

Date	Time	Blood Pressure		Pulse Heart Rate	Medication
		Systolic Top Number	Diastolic Bottom Number		
		/			
		/			
		/			
		/			
		/			
		/			
		/			
		/			

Blood Pressure Category	Systolic Top Number	Diastolic Bottom Number
Normal	Less than 120	Less than 80
Elevated	120 - 129	Less than 80
High Blood Pressure (Stage 1)	130 - 139	80-89
High Blood Pressure (Stage 2)	140 or higher	90 or higher
Hypertensive Crisis (Seek Emergency Care)	Higher than 180	Higher than 120

Blood Pressure Log

Month ____________ **Year** __________ **Weight** _________

Date	Time	Blood Pressure Systolic Top Number	Diastolic Bottom Number	Pulse Heart Rate	Medication
		/			
		/			
		/			
		/			
		/			
		/			
		/			
		/			
		/			
		/			
		/			

Notes

Blood Pressure Log

Month ___________ Year _________ Weight ________

Date	Time	Blood Pressure Systolic Top Number	Blood Pressure Diastolic Bottom Number	Pulse Heart Rate	Medication
		/			
		/			
		/			
		/			
		/			
		/			
		/			
		/			

Blood Pressure Category	Systolic Top Number	Diastolic Bottom Number
Normal	Less than 120	Less than 80
Elevated	120 - 129	Less than 80
High Blood Pressure (Stage 1)	130 - 139	80-89
High Blood Pressure (Stage 2)	140 or higher	90 or higher
Hypertensive Crisis (Seek Emergency Care)	Higher than 180	Higher than 120

Blood Pressure Log

Month ____________ **Year** __________ **Weight** ________

Date	Time	Blood Pressure: Systolic Top Number	Blood Pressure: Diastolic Bottom Number	Pulse Heart Rate	Medication
		/			
		/			
		/			
		/			
		/			
		/			
		/			
		/			
		/			
		/			
		/			

Notes

Blood Pressure Log

Month ____________ Year __________ Weight _________

Date	Time	Blood Pressure		Pulse Heart Rate	Medication
		Systolic Top Number	Diastolic Bottom Number		
		/			
		/			
		/			
		/			
		/			
		/			
		/			
		/			

Blood Pressure Category	Systolic Top Number	Diastolic Bottom Number
Normal	Less than 120	Less than 80
Elevated	120 - 129	Less than 80
High Blood Pressure (Stage 1)	130 - 139	80-89
High Blood Pressure (Stage 2)	140 or higher	90 or higher
Hypertensive Crisis (Seek Emergency Care)	Higher than 180	Higher than 120

Blood Pressure Log

Month ____________ **Year** ____________ **Weight** ____________

Date	Time	Blood Pressure		Pulse Heart Rate	Medication
		Systolic Top Number	Diastolic Bottom Number		
		/			
		/			
		/			
		/			
		/			
		/			
		/			
		/			
		/			
		/			
		/			

Notes

Blood Pressure Log

Month ____________ Year __________ Weight _________

Date	Time	Blood Pressure Systolic Top Number	Blood Pressure Diastolic Bottom Number	Pulse Heart Rate	Medication
		/			
		/			
		/			
		/			
		/			
		/			
		/			
		/			

Blood Pressure Category	Systolic Top Number	Diastolic Bottom Number
Normal	Less than 120	Less than 80
Elevated	120 - 129	Less than 80
High Blood Pressure (Stage 1)	130 - 139	80-89
High Blood Pressure (Stage 2)	140 or higher	90 or higher
Hypertensive Crisis (Seek Emergency Care)	Higher than 180	Higher than 120

Blood Pressure Log

Month ____________ **Year** __________ **Weight** _________

Date	Time	Blood Pressure: Systolic (Top Number)	Blood Pressure: Diastolic (Bottom Number)	Pulse (Heart Rate)	Medication
		/			
		/			
		/			
		/			
		/			
		/			
		/			
		/			
		/			
		/			
		/			

Notes

Blood Pressure Log

Month ____________ Year __________ Weight _________

Date	Time	Blood Pressure		Pulse Heart Rate	Medication
		Systolic Top Number	Diastolic Bottom Number		
		/			
		/			
		/			
		/			
		/			
		/			
		/			
		/			

Blood Pressure Category	Systolic Top Number	Diastolic Bottom Number
Normal	Less than 120	Less than 80
Elevated	120 - 129	Less than 80
High Blood Pressure (Stage 1)	130 - 139	80-89
High Blood Pressure (Stage 2)	140 or higher	90 or higher
Hypertensive Crisis (Seek Emergency Care)	Higher than 180	Higher than 120

Blood Pressure Log

Month ______________ **Year** __________ **Weight** __________

Date	Time	Blood Pressure: Systolic Top Number	Blood Pressure: Diastolic Bottom Number	Pulse Heart Rate	Medication
		/			
		/			
		/			
		/			
		/			
		/			
		/			
		/			
		/			
		/			
		/			

Notes

Blood Pressure Log

Month ____________ Year __________ Weight _________

Date	Time	Blood Pressure: Systolic Top Number	Blood Pressure: Diastolic Bottom Number	Pulse Heart Rate	Medication
		/			
		/			
		/			
		/			
		/			
		/			
		/			
		/			

Blood Pressure Category	Systolic Top Number	Diastolic Bottom Number
Normal	Less than 120	Less than 80
Elevated	120 - 129	Less than 80
High Blood Pressure (Stage 1)	130 - 139	80-89
High Blood Pressure (Stage 2)	140 or higher	90 or higher
Hypertensive Crisis (Seek Emergency Care)	Higher than 180	Higher than 120

Blood Pressure Log

Month ____________ Year ___________ Weight _________

Date	Time	Blood Pressure Systolic Top Number	Blood Pressure Diastolic Bottom Number	Pulse Heart Rate	Medication
		/			
		/			
		/			
		/			
		/			
		/			
		/			
		/			
		/			
		/			
		/			

Notes

Blood Pressure Log

Month ____________ Year __________ Weight _________

Date	Time	Blood Pressure Systolic Top Number	Blood Pressure Diastolic Bottom Number	Pulse Heart Rate	Medication
		/			
		/			
		/			
		/			
		/			
		/			
		/			
		/			

Blood Pressure Category	Systolic Top Number	Diastolic Bottom Number
Normal	Less than 120	Less than 80
Elevated	120 - 129	Less than 80
High Blood Pressure (Stage 1)	130 - 139	80-89
High Blood Pressure (Stage 2)	140 or higher	90 or higher
Hypertensive Crisis (Seek Emergency Care)	Higher than 180	Higher than 120

Blood Pressure Log

Month ____________ **Year** __________ **Weight** _________

Date	Time	Blood Pressure		Pulse Heart Rate	Medication
		Systolic Top Number	Diastolic Bottom Number		
		/			
		/			
		/			
		/			
		/			
		/			
		/			
		/			
		/			
		/			
		/			

Notes

Blood Pressure Log

Month ____________ Year __________ Weight _________

Date	Time	Blood Pressure: Systolic Top Number	Blood Pressure: Diastolic Bottom Number	Pulse Heart Rate	Medication
		/			
		/			
		/			
		/			
		/			
		/			
		/			
		/			

Blood Pressure Category	Systolic Top Number	Diastolic Bottom Number
Normal	Less than 120	Less than 80
Elevated	120 - 129	Less than 80
High Blood Pressure (Stage 1)	130 - 139	80-89
High Blood Pressure (Stage 2)	140 or higher	90 or higher
Hypertensive Crisis (Seek Emergency Care)	Higher than 180	Higher than 120

Blood Pressure Log

Month ____________ **Year** __________ **Weight** __________

Date	Time	Blood Pressure: Systolic Top Number	Blood Pressure: Diastolic Bottom Number	Pulse Heart Rate	Medication
		/			
		/			
		/			
		/			
		/			
		/			
		/			
		/			
		/			
		/			
		/			

Notes

Blood Pressure Log

Month ____________ Year __________ Weight _________

Date	Time	Blood Pressure Systolic Top Number	 Diastolic Bottom Number	Pulse Heart Rate	Medication
		/			
		/			
		/			
		/			
		/			
		/			
		/			
		/			

Blood Pressure Category	Systolic Top Number	Diastolic Bottom Number
Normal	Less than 120	Less than 80
Elevated	120 - 129	Less than 80
High Blood Pressure (Stage 1)	130 - 139	80-89
High Blood Pressure (Stage 2)	140 or higher	90 or higher
Hypertensive Crisis (Seek Emergency Care)	Higher than 180	Higher than 120

Blood Pressure Log

Month ____________ **Year** __________ **Weight** _________

Date	Time	Blood Pressure Systolic Top Number	 Diastolic Bottom Number	Pulse Heart Rate	Medication
		/			
		/			
		/			
		/			
		/			
		/			
		/			
		/			
		/			
		/			
		/			

Notes

Blood Pressure Log

Month ____________ Year __________ Weight _________

Date	Time	Blood Pressure: Systolic Top Number	Blood Pressure: Diastolic Bottom Number	Pulse Heart Rate	Medication
		/			
		/			
		/			
		/			
		/			
		/			
		/			
		/			

Blood Pressure Category	Systolic Top Number	Diastolic Bottom Number
Normal	Less than 120	Less than 80
Elevated	120 - 129	Less than 80
High Blood Pressure (Stage 1)	130 - 139	80-89
High Blood Pressure (Stage 2)	140 or higher	90 or higher
Hypertensive Crisis (Seek Emergency Care)	Higher than 180	Higher than 120

Blood Pressure Log

Month ____________ Year __________ Weight _________

Date	Time	Blood Pressure Systolic Top Number / Diastolic Bottom Number	Pulse Heart Rate	Medication
		/		
		/		
		/		
		/		
		/		
		/		
		/		
		/		
		/		
		/		
		/		

Notes

Blood Pressure Log

Month ____________ Year __________ Weight _________

Date	Time	Blood Pressure		Pulse	Medication
		Systolic Top Number	Diastolic Bottom Number	Pulse Heart Rate	
		/			
		/			
		/			
		/			
		/			
		/			
		/			
		/			

Blood Pressure Category	Systolic Top Number	Diastolic Bottom Number
Normal	Less than 120	Less than 80
Elevated	120 - 129	Less than 80
High Blood Pressure (Stage 1)	130 - 139	80-89
High Blood Pressure (Stage 2)	140 or higher	90 or higher
Hypertensive Crisis (Seek Emergency Care)	Higher than 180	Higher than 120

Blood Pressure Log

Month ____________ **Year** __________ **Weight** ________

Date	Time	Blood Pressure Systolic Top Number	Blood Pressure Diastolic Bottom Number	Pulse Heart Rate	Medication
		/			
		/			
		/			
		/			
		/			
		/			
		/			
		/			
		/			
		/			
		/			

Notes

Blood Pressure Log

Month ___________ Year _________ Weight ________

Date	Time	Blood Pressure: Systolic Top Number	Blood Pressure: Diastolic Bottom Number	Pulse Heart Rate	Medication
		/			
		/			
		/			
		/			
		/			
		/			
		/			
		/			

Blood Pressure Category	Systolic Top Number	Diastolic Bottom Number
Normal	Less than 120	Less than 80
Elevated	120 - 129	Less than 80
High Blood Pressure (Stage 1)	130 - 139	80-89
High Blood Pressure (Stage 2)	140 or higher	90 or higher
Hypertensive Crisis (Seek Emergency Care)	Higher than 180	Higher than 120

Blood Pressure Log

Month ____________ **Year** __________ **Weight** _________

Date	Time	Blood Pressure: Systolic Top Number	Blood Pressure: Diastolic Bottom Number	Pulse Heart Rate	Medication
		/			
		/			
		/			
		/			
		/			
		/			
		/			
		/			
		/			
		/			
		/			

Notes

Blood Pressure Log

Month ____________ Year __________ Weight __________

Date	Time	Blood Pressure Systolic Top Number	 Diastolic Bottom Number	Pulse Heart Rate	Medication
		/			
		/			
		/			
		/			
		/			
		/			
		/			
		/			

Blood Pressure Category	Systolic Top Number	Diastolic Bottom Number
Normal	Less than 120	Less than 80
Elevated	120 - 129	Less than 80
High Blood Pressure (Stage 1)	130 - 139	80-89
High Blood Pressure (Stage 2)	140 or higher	90 or higher
Hypertensive Crisis (Seek Emergency Care)	Higher than 180	Higher than 120

Blood Pressure Log

Month ____________ **Year** __________ **Weight** ________

Date	Time	Blood Pressure Systolic Top Number	 Diastolic Bottom Number	Pulse Heart Rate	Medication
		/			
		/			
		/			
		/			
		/			
		/			
		/			
		/			
		/			
		/			
		/			

Notes

Blood Pressure Log

Month ____________ Year __________ Weight _________

Date	Time	Blood Pressure		Pulse Heart Rate	Medication
		Systolic Top Number	Diastolic Bottom Number		
		/			
		/			
		/			
		/			
		/			
		/			
		/			
		/			

Blood Pressure Category	Systolic Top Number	Diastolic Bottom Number
Normal	Less than 120	Less than 80
Elevated	120 - 129	Less than 80
High Blood Pressure (Stage 1)	130 - 139	80-89
High Blood Pressure (Stage 2)	140 or higher	90 or higher
Hypertensive Crisis (Seek Emergency Care)	Higher than 180	Higher than 120

Blood Pressure Log

Month ____________ **Year** __________ **Weight** _________

Date	Time	Blood Pressure: Systolic Top Number	Blood Pressure: Diastolic Bottom Number	Pulse Heart Rate	Medication
		/			
		/			
		/			
		/			
		/			
		/			
		/			
		/			
		/			
		/			
		/			

Notes

Blood Pressure Log

Month ____________ Year __________ Weight _________

Date	Time	Blood Pressure: Systolic Top Number / Diastolic Bottom Number	Pulse Heart Rate	Medication
		/		
		/		
		/		
		/		
		/		
		/		
		/		
		/		

Blood Pressure Category	Systolic Top Number	Diastolic Bottom Number
Normal	Less than 120	Less than 80
Elevated	120 - 129	Less than 80
High Blood Pressure (Stage 1)	130 - 139	80-89
High Blood Pressure (Stage 2)	140 or higher	90 or higher
Hypertensive Crisis (Seek Emergency Care)	Higher than 180	Higher than 120

Blood Pressure Log

Month ____________ **Year** __________ **Weight** ________

Date	Time	Blood Pressure Systolic Top Number	Blood Pressure Diastolic Bottom Number	Pulse Heart Rate	Medication
		/			
		/			
		/			
		/			
		/			
		/			
		/			
		/			
		/			
		/			
		/			

Notes

Blood Pressure Log

Month __________ Year __________ Weight __________

Date	Time	Blood Pressure Systolic Top Number	Diastolic Bottom Number	Pulse Heart Rate	Medication
		/			
		/			
		/			
		/			
		/			
		/			
		/			
		/			

Blood Pressure Category	Systolic Top Number	Diastolic Bottom Number
Normal	Less than 120	Less than 80
Elevated	120 - 129	Less than 80
High Blood Pressure (Stage 1)	130 - 139	80-89
High Blood Pressure (Stage 2)	140 or higher	90 or higher
Hypertensive Crisis (Seek Emergency Care)	Higher than 180	Higher than 120

Blood Pressure Log

Month ____________ **Year** __________ **Weight** ________

Date	Time	Blood Pressure: Systolic Top Number	Blood Pressure: Diastolic Bottom Number	Pulse Heart Rate	Medication
		/			
		/			
		/			
		/			
		/			
		/			
		/			
		/			
		/			
		/			
		/			

Notes

Blood Pressure Log

Month ____________ Year ____________ Weight ____________

Date	Time	Blood Pressure Systolic Top Number	 Diastolic Bottom Number	Pulse Heart Rate	Medication
		/			
		/			
		/			
		/			
		/			
		/			
		/			
		/			

Blood Pressure Category	Systolic Top Number	Diastolic Bottom Number
Normal	Less than 120	Less than 80
Elevated	120 - 129	Less than 80
High Blood Pressure (Stage 1)	130 - 139	80-89
High Blood Pressure (Stage 2)	140 or higher	90 or higher
Hypertensive Crisis (Seek Emergency Care)	Higher than 180	Higher than 120

Blood Pressure Log

Month ____________ **Year** __________ **Weight** ________

Date	Time	Blood Pressure		Pulse	Medication
		Systolic Top Number	**Diastolic** Bottom Number	**Pulse** Heart Rate	
		/			
		/			
		/			
		/			
		/			
		/			
		/			
		/			
		/			
		/			
		/			

Notes

Blood Pressure Log

Month ____________ Year __________ Weight _________

Date	Time	Blood Pressure: <u>Systolic</u> Top Number	Blood Pressure: <u>Diastolic</u> Bottom Number	<u>Pulse</u> Heart Rate	Medication
		/			
		/			
		/			
		/			
		/			
		/			
		/			
		/			

Blood Pressure Category	Systolic Top Number	Diastolic Bottom Number
Normal	Less than 120	Less than 80
Elevated	120 - 129	Less than 80
High Blood Pressure (Stage 1)	130 - 139	80-89
High Blood Pressure (Stage 2)	140 or higher	90 or higher
Hypertensive Crisis (Seek Emergency Care)	Higher than 180	Higher than 120

Blood Pressure Log

Month ____________ **Year** ___________ **Weight** _________

Date	Time	Blood Pressure Systolic Top Number	Blood Pressure Diastolic Bottom Number	Pulse Heart Rate	Medication
		/			
		/			
		/			
		/			
		/			
		/			
		/			
		/			
		/			
		/			
		/			

Notes

Blood Pressure Log

Month ____________ Year __________ Weight _________

Date	Time	Blood Pressure: Systolic Top Number	Blood Pressure: Diastolic Bottom Number	Pulse Heart Rate	Medication
		/			
		/			
		/			
		/			
		/			
		/			
		/			
		/			

Blood Pressure Category	Systolic Top Number	Diastolic Bottom Number
Normal	Less than 120	Less than 80
Elevated	120 - 129	Less than 80
High Blood Pressure (Stage 1)	130 - 139	80-89
High Blood Pressure (Stage 2)	140 or higher	90 or higher
Hypertensive Crisis (Seek Emergency Care)	Higher than 180	Higher than 120

Blood Pressure Log

Month ____________ **Year** __________ **Weight** ________

Date	Time	Blood Pressure Systolic Top Number	Diastolic Bottom Number	Pulse Heart Rate	Medication
		/			
		/			
		/			
		/			
		/			
		/			
		/			
		/			
		/			
		/			
		/			

Notes

Blood Pressure Log

Month ____________ Year __________ Weight _________

Date	Time	Blood Pressure Systolic Top Number	 Diastolic Bottom Number	Pulse Heart Rate	Medication
		/			
		/			
		/			
		/			
		/			
		/			
		/			
		/			

Blood Pressure Category	Systolic Top Number	Diastolic Bottom Number
Normal	Less than 120	Less than 80
Elevated	120 - 129	Less than 80
High Blood Pressure (Stage 1)	130 - 139	80-89
High Blood Pressure (Stage 2)	140 or higher	90 or higher
Hypertensive Crisis (Seek Emergency Care)	Higher than 180	Higher than 120

Blood Pressure Log

Month ______________ **Year** __________ **Weight** __________

Date	Time	Blood Pressure Systolic Top Number	Blood Pressure Diastolic Bottom Number	Pulse Heart Rate	Medication
		/			
		/			
		/			
		/			
		/			
		/			
		/			
		/			
		/			
		/			
		/			

Notes

Blood Pressure Log

Month __________ Year __________ Weight __________

Date	Time	Blood Pressure		Pulse	Medication
		Systolic Top Number	Diastolic Bottom Number	Pulse Heart Rate	
		/			
		/			
		/			
		/			
		/			
		/			
		/			
		/			

Blood Pressure Category	Systolic Top Number	Diastolic Bottom Number
Normal	Less than 120	Less than 80
Elevated	120 - 129	Less than 80
High Blood Pressure (Stage 1)	130 - 139	80-89
High Blood Pressure (Stage 2)	140 or higher	90 or higher
Hypertensive Crisis (Seek Emergency Care)	Higher than 180	Higher than 120

Blood Pressure Log

Month ____________ **Year** __________ **Weight** _________

Date	Time	Blood Pressure Systolic Top Number	 Diastolic Bottom Number	Pulse Heart Rate	Medication
		/			
		/			
		/			
		/			
		/			
		/			
		/			
		/			
		/			
		/			
		/			

Notes

Blood Pressure Log

Month __________ Year __________ Weight __________

Date	Time	Blood Pressure Systolic Top Number	Blood Pressure Diastolic Bottom Number	Pulse Heart Rate	Medication
		/			
		/			
		/			
		/			
		/			
		/			
		/			
		/			

Blood Pressure Category	Systolic Top Number	Diastolic Bottom Number
Normal	Less than 120	Less than 80
Elevated	120 - 129	Less than 80
High Blood Pressure (Stage 1)	130 - 139	80-89
High Blood Pressure (Stage 2)	140 or higher	90 or higher
Hypertensive Crisis (Seek Emergency Care)	Higher than 180	Higher than 120

Blood Pressure Log

Month ____________ Year __________ Weight _________

Date	Time	Blood Pressure Systolic Top Number	Blood Pressure Diastolic Bottom Number	Pulse Heart Rate	Medication
		/			
		/			
		/			
		/			
		/			
		/			
		/			
		/			
		/			
		/			
		/			

Notes

Blood Pressure Log

Month ____________ Year __________ Weight _________

Date	Time	Blood Pressure		Pulse Heart Rate	Medication
		Systolic Top Number	Diastolic Bottom Number		
		/			
		/			
		/			
		/			
		/			
		/			
		/			
		/			

Blood Pressure Category	Systolic Top Number	Diastolic Bottom Number
Normal	Less than 120	Less than 80
Elevated	120 - 129	Less than 80
High Blood Pressure (Stage 1)	130 - 139	80-89
High Blood Pressure (Stage 2)	140 or higher	90 or higher
Hypertensive Crisis (Seek Emergency Care)	Higher than 180	Higher than 120

Blood Pressure Log

Month ____________ **Year** __________ **Weight** ________

Date	Time	Blood Pressure: Systolic Top Number	Blood Pressure: Diastolic Bottom Number	Pulse Heart Rate	Medication
		/			
		/			
		/			
		/			
		/			
		/			
		/			
		/			
		/			
		/			
		/			

Notes

Blood Pressure Log

Month ____________ Year __________ Weight _________

Date	Time	Blood Pressure Systolic Top Number	Blood Pressure Diastolic Bottom Number	Pulse Heart Rate	Medication
		/			
		/			
		/			
		/			
		/			
		/			
		/			
		/			

Blood Pressure Category	Systolic Top Number	Diastolic Bottom Number
Normal	Less than 120	Less than 80
Elevated	120 - 129	Less than 80
High Blood Pressure (Stage 1)	130 - 139	80-89
High Blood Pressure (Stage 2)	140 or higher	90 or higher
Hypertensive Crisis (Seek Emergency Care)	Higher than 180	Higher than 120

Blood Pressure Log

Month ____________ **Year** __________ **Weight** ________

Date	Time	Blood Pressure Systolic Top Number	Diastolic Bottom Number	Pulse Heart Rate	Medication
		/			
		/			
		/			
		/			
		/			
		/			
		/			
		/			
		/			
		/			
		/			

Notes

Blood Pressure Log

Month ____________ Year __________ Weight _________

Date	Time	Blood Pressure: Systolic Top Number	Blood Pressure: Diastolic Bottom Number	Pulse Heart Rate	Medication
		/			
		/			
		/			
		/			
		/			
		/			
		/			
		/			

Blood Pressure Category	Systolic Top Number	Diastolic Bottom Number
Normal	Less than 120	Less than 80
Elevated	120 - 129	Less than 80
High Blood Pressure (Stage 1)	130 - 139	80-89
High Blood Pressure (Stage 2)	140 or higher	90 or higher
Hypertensive Crisis (Seek Emergency Care)	Higher than 180	Higher than 120

Blood Pressure Log

Month ____________ **Year** __________ **Weight** _________

Date	Time	Blood Pressure Systolic Top Number	Blood Pressure Diastolic Bottom Number	Pulse Heart Rate	Medication
		/			
		/			
		/			
		/			
		/			
		/			
		/			
		/			
		/			
		/			
		/			

Notes

Blood Pressure Log

Month ____________ Year __________ Weight _________

Date	Time	Blood Pressure Systolic Top Number	Blood Pressure Diastolic Bottom Number	Pulse Heart Rate	Medication
		/			
		/			
		/			
		/			
		/			
		/			
		/			
		/			

Blood Pressure Category	Systolic Top Number	Diastolic Bottom Number
Normal	Less than 120	Less than 80
Elevated	120 - 129	Less than 80
High Blood Pressure (Stage 1)	130 - 139	80-89
High Blood Pressure (Stage 2)	140 or higher	90 or higher
Hypertensive Crisis (Seek Emergency Care)	Higher than 180	Higher than 120

Blood Pressure Log

Month ____________ **Year** __________ **Weight** _________

Date	Time	Blood Pressure: Systolic Top Number	Blood Pressure: Diastolic Bottom Number	Pulse Heart Rate	Medication
		/			
		/			
		/			
		/			
		/			
		/			
		/			
		/			
		/			
		/			
		/			

Notes

Blood Pressure Log

Month ____________ Year __________ Weight _________

Date	Time	Blood Pressure: Systolic Top Number	Blood Pressure: Diastolic Bottom Number	Pulse Heart Rate	Medication
		/			
		/			
		/			
		/			
		/			
		/			
		/			
		/			

Blood Pressure Category	Systolic Top Number	Diastolic Bottom Number
Normal	Less than 120	Less than 80
Elevated	120 - 129	Less than 80
High Blood Pressure (Stage 1)	130 - 139	80-89
High Blood Pressure (Stage 2)	140 or higher	90 or higher
Hypertensive Crisis (Seek Emergency Care)	Higher than 180	Higher than 120

Blood Pressure Log

Month ____________ **Year** __________ **Weight** __________

Date	Time	Blood Pressure Systolic Top Number	Blood Pressure Diastolic Bottom Number	Pulse Heart Rate	Medication
		/			
		/			
		/			
		/			
		/			
		/			
		/			
		/			
		/			
		/			
		/			

Notes

Blood Pressure Log

Month ____________ Year __________ Weight _________

Date	Time	Blood Pressure: Systolic Top Number	Blood Pressure: Diastolic Bottom Number	Pulse Heart Rate	Medication
		/			
		/			
		/			
		/			
		/			
		/			
		/			
		/			

Blood Pressure Category	Systolic Top Number	Diastolic Bottom Number
Normal	Less than 120	Less than 80
Elevated	120 - 129	Less than 80
High Blood Pressure (Stage 1)	130 - 139	80-89
High Blood Pressure (Stage 2)	140 or higher	90 or higher
Hypertensive Crisis (Seek Emergency Care)	Higher than 180	Higher than 120

Blood Pressure Log

Month ____________ **Year** __________ **Weight** ________

Date	Time	Blood Pressure Systolic Top Number	 Diastolic Bottom Number	Pulse Heart Rate	Medication
		/			
		/			
		/			
		/			
		/			
		/			
		/			
		/			
		/			
		/			
		/			

Notes

Blood Pressure Log

Month ____________ Year __________ Weight _________

Date	Time	Blood Pressure: Systolic Top Number	Blood Pressure: Diastolic Bottom Number	Pulse Heart Rate	Medication
		/			
		/			
		/			
		/			
		/			
		/			
		/			
		/			

Blood Pressure Category	Systolic Top Number	Diastolic Bottom Number
Normal	Less than 120	Less than 80
Elevated	120 - 129	Less than 80
High Blood Pressure (Stage 1)	130 - 139	80-89
High Blood Pressure (Stage 2)	140 or higher	90 or higher
Hypertensive Crisis (Seek Emergency Care)	Higher than 180	Higher than 120

Blood Pressure Log

Month ____________ **Year** __________ **Weight** _________

Date	Time	Blood Pressure Systolic Top Number	 Diastolic Bottom Number	Pulse Heart Rate	Medication
		/			
		/			
		/			
		/			
		/			
		/			
		/			
		/			
		/			
		/			
		/			

Notes

Blood Pressure Log

Month ____________ Year __________ Weight _________

Date	Time	Blood Pressure		Pulse	Medication
		Systolic Top Number	Diastolic Bottom Number	Heart Rate	
		/			
		/			
		/			
		/			
		/			
		/			
		/			
		/			

Blood Pressure Category	Systolic Top Number	Diastolic Bottom Number
Normal	Less than 120	Less than 80
Elevated	120 - 129	Less than 80
High Blood Pressure (Stage 1)	130 - 139	80-89
High Blood Pressure (Stage 2)	140 or higher	90 or higher
Hypertensive Crisis (Seek Emergency Care)	Higher than 180	Higher than 120

Blood Pressure Log

Month ____________ **Year** __________ **Weight** __________

Date	Time	Blood Pressure		Pulse	Medication
		Systolic Top Number	**Diastolic** Bottom Number	**Pulse** Heart Rate	
		/			
		/			
		/			
		/			
		/			
		/			
		/			
		/			
		/			
		/			
		/			

Notes

Blood Pressure Log

Month ____________ Year __________ Weight _________

Date	Time	Blood Pressure: Systolic Top Number	Blood Pressure: Diastolic Bottom Number	Pulse Heart Rate	Medication
		/			
		/			
		/			
		/			
		/			
		/			
		/			
		/			

Blood Pressure Category	Systolic Top Number	Diastolic Bottom Number
Normal	Less than 120	Less than 80
Elevated	120 - 129	Less than 80
High Blood Pressure (Stage 1)	130 - 139	80-89
High Blood Pressure (Stage 2)	140 or higher	90 or higher
Hypertensive Crisis (Seek Emergency Care)	Higher than 180	Higher than 120

Blood Pressure Log

Month ____________ Year __________ Weight _________

Date	Time	Blood Pressure Systolic Top Number	Blood Pressure Diastolic Bottom Number	Pulse Heart Rate	Medication
		/			
		/			
		/			
		/			
		/			
		/			
		/			
		/			
		/			
		/			
		/			

Notes

Blood Pressure Log

Month ____________ Year __________ Weight _________

Date	Time	Blood Pressure Systolic Top Number / Diastolic Bottom Number		Pulse Heart Rate	Medication
		/			
		/			
		/			
		/			
		/			
		/			
		/			
		/			

Blood Pressure Category	Systolic Top Number	Diastolic Bottom Number
Normal	Less than 120	Less than 80
Elevated	120 - 129	Less than 80
High Blood Pressure (Stage 1)	130 - 139	80-89
High Blood Pressure (Stage 2)	140 or higher	90 or higher
Hypertensive Crisis (Seek Emergency Care)	Higher than 180	Higher than 120

Blood Pressure Log

Month ____________ **Year** __________ **Weight** ________

Date	Time	Blood Pressure: Systolic Top Number	Blood Pressure: Diastolic Bottom Number	Pulse Heart Rate	Medication
		/			
		/			
		/			
		/			
		/			
		/			
		/			
		/			
		/			
		/			
		/			

Notes

Blood Pressure Log

Month __________ **Year** __________ **Weight** __________

Date	Time	Blood Pressure Systolic Top Number	 Diastolic Bottom Number	Pulse Heart Rate	Medication
		/			
		/			
		/			
		/			
		/			
		/			
		/			
		/			

Blood Pressure Category	Systolic Top Number	Diastolic Bottom Number
Normal	Less than 120	Less than 80
Elevated	120 - 129	Less than 80
High Blood Pressure (Stage 1)	130 - 139	80-89
High Blood Pressure (Stage 2)	140 or higher	90 or higher
Hypertensive Crisis (Seek Emergency Care)	Higher than 180	Higher than 120

Blood Pressure Log

Month ____________ **Year** __________ **Weight** _________

Date	Time	Blood Pressure: Systolic Top Number	Blood Pressure: Diastolic Bottom Number	Pulse Heart Rate	Medication
		/			
		/			
		/			
		/			
		/			
		/			
		/			
		/			
		/			
		/			
		/			

Notes

Blood Pressure Log

Month ____________ Year __________ Weight _________

Date	Time	Blood Pressure: Systolic (Top Number)	Blood Pressure: Diastolic (Bottom Number)	Pulse (Heart Rate)	Medication
		/			
		/			
		/			
		/			
		/			
		/			
		/			
		/			

Blood Pressure Category	Systolic Top Number	Diastolic Bottom Number
Normal	Less than 120	Less than 80
Elevated	120 - 129	Less than 80
High Blood Pressure (Stage 1)	130 - 139	80-89
High Blood Pressure (Stage 2)	140 or higher	90 or higher
Hypertensive Crisis (Seek Emergency Care)	Higher than 180	Higher than 120

Blood Pressure Log

Month ____________ **Year** __________ **Weight** ________

Date	Time	Blood Pressure Systolic Top Number	Blood Pressure Diastolic Bottom Number	Pulse Heart Rate	Medication
		/			
		/			
		/			
		/			
		/			
		/			
		/			
		/			
		/			
		/			
		/			

Notes

Blood Pressure Log

Month ____________ Year __________ Weight _________

Date	Time	Blood Pressure: Systolic Top Number	Blood Pressure: Diastolic Bottom Number	Pulse Heart Rate	Medication
		/			
		/			
		/			
		/			
		/			
		/			
		/			
		/			

Blood Pressure Category	Systolic Top Number	Diastolic Bottom Number
Normal	Less than 120	Less than 80
Elevated	120 - 129	Less than 80
High Blood Pressure (Stage 1)	130 - 139	80-89
High Blood Pressure (Stage 2)	140 or higher	90 or higher
Hypertensive Crisis (Seek Emergency Care)	Higher than 180	Higher than 120

Blood Pressure Log

Month ____________ **Year** __________ **Weight** __________

Date	Time	Blood Pressure Systolic Top Number	Blood Pressure Diastolic Bottom Number	Pulse Heart Rate	Medication
		/			
		/			
		/			
		/			
		/			
		/			
		/			
		/			
		/			
		/			
		/			

Notes

Blood Pressure Log

Month ____________ Year __________ Weight _________

Date	Time	Blood Pressure		Pulse Heart Rate	Medication
		Systolic Top Number	Diastolic Bottom Number		
		/			
		/			
		/			
		/			
		/			
		/			
		/			
		/			

Blood Pressure Category	Systolic Top Number	Diastolic Bottom Number
Normal	Less than 120	Less than 80
Elevated	120 - 129	Less than 80
High Blood Pressure (Stage 1)	130 - 139	80-89
High Blood Pressure (Stage 2)	140 or higher	90 or higher
Hypertensive Crisis (Seek Emergency Care)	Higher than 180	Higher than 120

Blood Pressure Log

Month ____________ **Year** __________ **Weight** _________

Date	Time	Blood Pressure Systolic Top Number	Blood Pressure Diastolic Bottom Number	Pulse Heart Rate	Medication
		/			
		/			
		/			
		/			
		/			
		/			
		/			
		/			
		/			
		/			
		/			

Notes

Blood Pressure Log

Month ____________ Year __________ Weight _________

Date	Time	Blood Pressure Systolic Top Number	Blood Pressure Diastolic Bottom Number	Pulse Heart Rate	Medication
		/			
		/			
		/			
		/			
		/			
		/			
		/			
		/			

Blood Pressure Category	Systolic Top Number	Diastolic Bottom Number
Normal	Less than 120	Less than 80
Elevated	120 - 129	Less than 80
High Blood Pressure (Stage 1)	130 - 139	80-89
High Blood Pressure (Stage 2)	140 or higher	90 or higher
Hypertensive Crisis (Seek Emergency Care)	Higher than 180	Higher than 120

Blood Pressure Log

Month ____________ **Year** __________ **Weight** _________

Date	Time	Blood Pressure Systolic Top Number	 Diastolic Bottom Number	Pulse Heart Rate	Medication
		/			
		/			
		/			
		/			
		/			
		/			
		/			
		/			
		/			
		/			
		/			

Notes

Blood Pressure Log

Month ____________ Year __________ Weight _________

Date	Time	Blood Pressure		Pulse	Medication
		Systolic Top Number	Diastolic Bottom Number	Heart Rate	
		/			
		/			
		/			
		/			
		/			
		/			
		/			
		/			

Blood Pressure Category	Systolic Top Number	Diastolic Bottom Number
Normal	Less than 120	Less than 80
Elevated	120 - 129	Less than 80
High Blood Pressure (Stage 1)	130 - 139	80-89
High Blood Pressure (Stage 2)	140 or higher	90 or higher
Hypertensive Crisis (Seek Emergency Care)	Higher than 180	Higher than 120

Blood Pressure Log

Month ____________ Year __________ Weight ________

Date	Time	Blood Pressure: Systolic (Top Number)	Blood Pressure: Diastolic (Bottom Number)	Pulse (Heart Rate)	Medication
		/			
		/			
		/			
		/			
		/			
		/			
		/			
		/			
		/			
		/			
		/			

Notes

Blood Pressure Log

Month ______________ Year ___________ Weight __________

Date	Time	Blood Pressure: Systolic (Top Number)	Blood Pressure: Diastolic (Bottom Number)	Pulse (Heart Rate)	Medication
		/			
		/			
		/			
		/			
		/			
		/			
		/			
		/			

Blood Pressure Category	Systolic Top Number	Diastolic Bottom Number
Normal	Less than 120	Less than 80
Elevated	120 - 129	Less than 80
High Blood Pressure (Stage 1)	130 - 139	80-89
High Blood Pressure (Stage 2)	140 or higher	90 or higher
Hypertensive Crisis (Seek Emergency Care)	Higher than 180	Higher than 120

Blood Pressure Log

Month ____________ **Year** __________ **Weight** __________

Date	Time	Blood Pressure Systolic Top Number	Diastolic Bottom Number	Pulse Heart Rate	Medication
		/			
		/			
		/			
		/			
		/			
		/			
		/			
		/			
		/			
		/			
		/			

Notes

Blood Pressure Log

Month ___________ Year _________ Weight ________

Date	Time	Blood Pressure Systolic Top Number	Blood Pressure Diastolic Bottom Number	Pulse Heart Rate	Medication
		/			
		/			
		/			
		/			
		/			
		/			
		/			
		/			

Blood Pressure Category	Systolic Top Number	Diastolic Bottom Number
Normal	Less than 120	Less than 80
Elevated	120 - 129	Less than 80
High Blood Pressure (Stage 1)	130 - 139	80-89
High Blood Pressure (Stage 2)	140 or higher	90 or higher
Hypertensive Crisis (Seek Emergency Care)	Higher than 180	Higher than 120

Blood Pressure Log

Month ____________ **Year** __________ **Weight** _________

Date	Time	Blood Pressure Systolic Top Number	 Diastolic Bottom Number	Pulse Heart Rate	Medication
		/			
		/			
		/			
		/			
		/			
		/			
		/			
		/			
		/			
		/			
		/			

Notes

Blood Pressure Log

Month ____________ Year __________ Weight _________

Date	Time	Blood Pressure: Systolic Top Number	Blood Pressure: Diastolic Bottom Number	Pulse Heart Rate	Medication
		/			
		/			
		/			
		/			
		/			
		/			
		/			
		/			

Blood Pressure Category	Systolic Top Number	Diastolic Bottom Number
Normal	Less than 120	Less than 80
Elevated	120 - 129	Less than 80
High Blood Pressure (Stage 1)	130 - 139	80-89
High Blood Pressure (Stage 2)	140 or higher	90 or higher
Hypertensive Crisis (Seek Emergency Care)	Higher than 180	Higher than 120

Blood Pressure Log

Month ____________ **Year** __________ **Weight** _________

Date	Time	Blood Pressure Systolic Top Number	 Diastolic Bottom Number	Pulse Heart Rate	Medication
		/			
		/			
		/			
		/			
		/			
		/			
		/			
		/			
		/			
		/			
		/			

Notes

Blood Pressure Log

Month ____________ **Year** __________ **Weight** _________

Date	Time	Blood Pressure: Systolic Top Number	Blood Pressure: Diastolic Bottom Number	Pulse Heart Rate	Medication
		/			
		/			
		/			
		/			
		/			
		/			
		/			
		/			

Blood Pressure Category	Systolic Top Number	Diastolic Bottom Number
Normal	Less than 120	Less than 80
Elevated	120 - 129	Less than 80
High Blood Pressure (Stage 1)	130 - 139	80-89
High Blood Pressure (Stage 2)	140 or higher	90 or higher
Hypertensive Crisis (Seek Emergency Care)	Higher than 180	Higher than 120

Blood Pressure Log

Month ______________ **Year** ____________ **Weight** ____________

Date	Time	Blood Pressure Systolic Top Number	Blood Pressure Diastolic Bottom Number	Pulse Heart Rate	Medication
		/			
		/			
		/			
		/			
		/			
		/			
		/			
		/			
		/			
		/			
		/			

Notes

Blood Pressure Log

Month ___________ Year _________ Weight ________

Date	Time	Blood Pressure: Systolic Top Number	Blood Pressure: Diastolic Bottom Number	Pulse Heart Rate	Medication
		/			
		/			
		/			
		/			
		/			
		/			
		/			
		/			

Blood Pressure Category	Systolic Top Number	Diastolic Bottom Number
Normal	Less than 120	Less than 80
Elevated	120 - 129	Less than 80
High Blood Pressure (Stage 1)	130 - 139	80-89
High Blood Pressure (Stage 2)	140 or higher	90 or higher
Hypertensive Crisis (Seek Emergency Care)	Higher than 180	Higher than 120

Blood Pressure Log

Month ____________ Year __________ Weight _________

Date	Time	Blood Pressure: Systolic Top Number	Blood Pressure: Diastolic Bottom Number	Pulse Heart Rate	Medication
		/			
		/			
		/			
		/			
		/			
		/			
		/			
		/			
		/			
		/			
		/			

Notes

Blood Pressure Log

Month ____________ Year __________ Weight _________

Date	Time	Blood Pressure		Pulse	Medication
		Systolic Top Number	Diastolic Bottom Number	Heart Rate	
		/			
		/			
		/			
		/			
		/			
		/			
		/			
		/			

Blood Pressure Category	Systolic Top Number	Diastolic Bottom Number
Normal	Less than 120	Less than 80
Elevated	120 - 129	Less than 80
High Blood Pressure (Stage 1)	130 - 139	80-89
High Blood Pressure (Stage 2)	140 or higher	90 or higher
Hypertensive Crisis (Seek Emergency Care)	Higher than 180	Higher than 120

Blood Pressure Log

Month ________ **Year** ________ **Weight** ________

Date	Time	Blood Pressure Systolic Top Number	Blood Pressure Diastolic Bottom Number	Pulse Heart Rate	Medication
		/			
		/			
		/			
		/			
		/			
		/			
		/			
		/			
		/			
		/			
		/			

Notes

Blood Pressure Log

Month ____________ Year __________ Weight _________

Date	Time	Blood Pressure: Systolic (Top Number)	Blood Pressure: Diastolic (Bottom Number)	Pulse (Heart Rate)	Medication
		/			
		/			
		/			
		/			
		/			
		/			
		/			
		/			

Blood Pressure Category	Systolic Top Number	Diastolic Bottom Number
Normal	Less than 120	Less than 80
Elevated	120 - 129	Less than 80
High Blood Pressure (Stage 1)	130 - 139	80-89
High Blood Pressure (Stage 2)	140 or higher	90 or higher
Hypertensive Crisis (Seek Emergency Care)	Higher than 180	Higher than 120

Blood Pressure Log

Month ____________ **Year** __________ **Weight** _________

Date	Time	Blood Pressure Systolic Top Number	 Diastolic Bottom Number	Pulse Heart Rate	Medication
		/			
		/			
		/			
		/			
		/			
		/			
		/			
		/			
		/			
		/			
		/			

Notes

Blood Pressure Log

Month ____________ Year __________ Weight _________

Date	Time	Blood Pressure: Systolic Top Number	Blood Pressure: Diastolic Bottom Number	Pulse Heart Rate	Medication
		/			
		/			
		/			
		/			
		/			
		/			
		/			
		/			

Blood Pressure Category	Systolic Top Number	Diastolic Bottom Number
Normal	Less than 120	Less than 80
Elevated	120 - 129	Less than 80
High Blood Pressure (Stage 1)	130 - 139	80-89
High Blood Pressure (Stage 2)	140 or higher	90 or higher
Hypertensive Crisis (Seek Emergency Care)	Higher than 180	Higher than 120

Blood Pressure Log

Month ______________ **Year** ___________ **Weight** __________

Date	Time	Blood Pressure Systolic Top Number	 Diastolic Bottom Number	Pulse Heart Rate	Medication
		/			
		/			
		/			
		/			
		/			
		/			
		/			
		/			
		/			
		/			
		/			

Notes

Blood Pressure Log

Month ____________ Year __________ Weight _________

Date	Time	Blood Pressure		Pulse	Medication
		Systolic Top Number	Diastolic Bottom Number	Pulse Heart Rate	
		/			
		/			
		/			
		/			
		/			
		/			
		/			
		/			

Blood Pressure Category	Systolic Top Number	Diastolic Bottom Number
Normal	Less than 120	Less than 80
Elevated	120 - 129	Less than 80
High Blood Pressure (Stage 1)	130 - 139	80-89
High Blood Pressure (Stage 2)	140 or higher	90 or higher
Hypertensive Crisis (Seek Emergency Care)	Higher than 180	Higher than 120

Blood Pressure Log

Month ____________ **Year** __________ **Weight** __________

Date	Time	Blood Pressure		Pulse	Medication
		Systolic Top Number	Diastolic Bottom Number	Heart Rate	
		/			
		/			
		/			
		/			
		/			
		/			
		/			
		/			
		/			
		/			
		/			

Notes

Blood Pressure Log

Month ____________ Year __________ Weight _________

Date	Time	Blood Pressure		Pulse	Medication
		Systolic Top Number	Diastolic Bottom Number	Heart Rate	
		/			
		/			
		/			
		/			
		/			
		/			
		/			
		/			

Blood Pressure Category	Systolic Top Number	Diastolic Bottom Number
Normal	Less than 120	Less than 80
Elevated	120 - 129	Less than 80
High Blood Pressure (Stage 1)	130 - 139	80-89
High Blood Pressure (Stage 2)	140 or higher	90 or higher
Hypertensive Crisis (Seek Emergency Care)	Higher than 180	Higher than 120

NOTES

Name:

NOTES

Name:

STAY ORGANIZED
STAY EMPOWERED

Want a FREE Healthy Meal Planner?

Get your free printable, plus health tips to help you stay on track.

Visit: www.mealplan.adalynnjames.com
Enter your name & email to download instantly!

Enjoying this logbook?
Your honest review helps others find this book and supports businesses like ours.

Please take a minute to leave a review on Amazon. We read every single one! Scan the QR code below.

https://bit.ly/BloodPressureBookReviews

— DigiMedical, by Adalynn James Publishing

Digi Medical

ADALYNN JAMES

Made in the USA
Monee, IL
04 November 2026

67379636R00066